Oppositional Defiant Disorders: Possible Treatment and How to Overcome it in Children.

By

Angela J. Howell.

INTRODUCTION

In a world where developmental issues take many forms, Oppositional Defiant Disorder (ODD) presents a daunting task for both children and carers. This book is a light of hope in the middle of a storm, giving insights into the complexity of ODD and practical advice on how to navigate its turbulent seas.

This book digs into the varied nature of ODD, revealing its underlying origins and analyzing the wide range of treatment approaches available. Each chapter, from therapeutic treatments to behavioral techniques, is intended to provide carers with the information and resources they need to help their children recover and become more resilient.

This book is more than simply a symptom management guide; it is a monument to the human spirit's tenacity and the transformational power of love and understanding. Join this journey of learning and empowerment as we face the difficulties of Oppositional Defiant Disorder and conquer it together.

CHAPTER 1: UNDERSTANDING OPPOSITIONAL DEFIANT DISORDER

1.1 DEFINITION

Oppositional defiant disorder is a form of behavioral disorder. It is most often diagnosed during childhood. Children with ODD exhibit uncooperative, belligerent, and aggressive behavior towards classmates, parents, teachers, and other authority figures. They are more upsetting to others than to themselves.

Oppositional defiant disorder (ODD) is a mental health illness characterized by a recurrent pattern of irritable/angry mood, defiant/argumentative behavior, or vindictiveness lasting at least 6 months. Although the specific etiology of ODD is unknown, biological, genetic, and environmental factors are all thought to have a role.

Children with chemical abnormalities in the brain, as well as those with a positive parental history of mental health issues, and those born to mothers who smoked during pregnancy, are at an especially high risk of having ODD.

Patients are often angry and violent, with rebellious, spiteful, and generally unfavorable attitudes towards persons of authority. They show little interest in following rules, exhibit temper tantrums, blame others for their misbehavior, and are easily irritated.

ODD may impact up to 16% of children and adolescents, and it is present in up to half of people with attention-deficit/hyperactivity disorder (ADHD). However, mood disorders such as bipolar disorder and depression, as well as other illnesses such as learning and language problems, have been linked to ODD.

What Causes ODD in Children?

Researchers are not sure what causes ODD. However, there are two basic hypotheses on why it occurs:

•**Developmental Theory:** This idea proposes that the difficulties begin when children are toddlers. Children and teenagers with ODD may have struggled to develop independence from a parent or other significant figure to whom they were emotionally bonded. Their behavior might be typical developmental concerns that extend beyond the toddler years.

•**Learning Theory** : This approach proposes that the negative symptoms of ODD are learnt attitudes. They replicate the impacts of negative reinforcement strategies employed by parents and others in positions of authority. The use of negative reinforcement promotes the child's ODD behaviors. This is because these behaviors enable the youngster to get what he or she desires: attention and a response from parents or others.

Which youngsters are at risk of ODD?

ODD is more prevalent in boys than in girls. Children with the following mental health disorders are more likely to develop ODD.

Mood or anxiety disorders.

Conduct disorder

Attention deficit and hyperactivity disorder (ADHD)

What Are The Symptoms Of ODD?

The majority of symptoms noticed in children and teenagers with ODD may also be found in other children without it. This is particularly true for youngsters between the ages of two and three, as well as those in their teens. Many youngsters tend to disobey, dispute with their parents, or challenge authority.

They may often act in this manner when they are weary, hungry, or agitated. However, among children and adolescents with ODD, these symptoms occur more often. They also disrupt learning and school adjustment. In certain situations, they can interfere with the child's interpersonal ties.

Symptoms of ODD may include:

•Having frequent temper outbursts.

•Arguing excessively with grownups

•Refusing to follow an adult's instructions

•Constantly questioning and refusing to obey regulations.

•Doing actions that irritate or offend people, even adults.

•Blaming others for the child's own misbehaviours or faults.

•Getting easily upset by people

•Frequently exhibiting a hostile attitude

•Speak brutally or unkindly

•Seeking vengeance or vindictiveness

These symptoms may resemble other mental health issues. Make sure your child visits his or her doctor for a diagnosis.

According to the fourth version of the Diagnostic and Statistical Manual (DSM-IV-TR) (now updated by DSM-5), a person must display four of the eight signs and symptoms to be diagnosed with ODD.

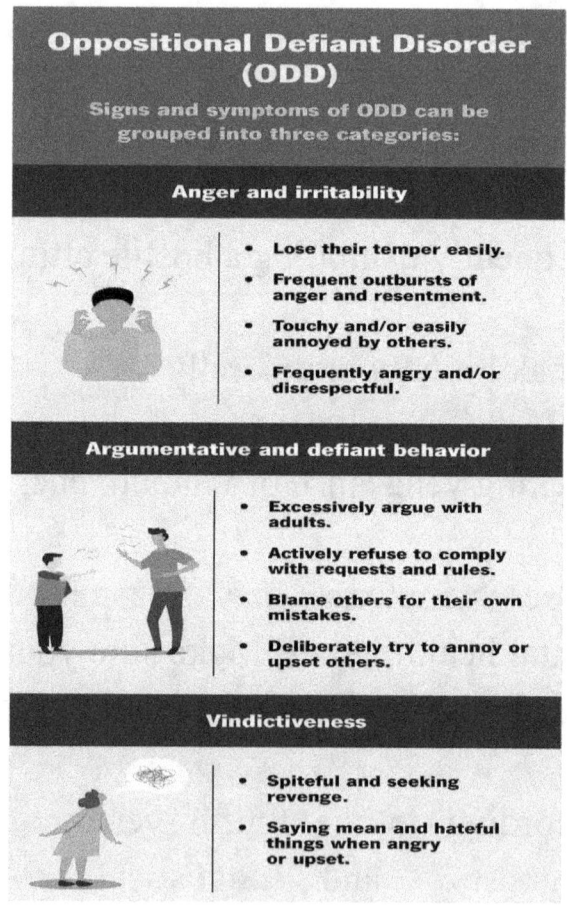

These behaviors are often aimed against an authority person, such as a teacher or parent. Although these behaviors are common among siblings, an ODD diagnosis requires observation with persons other than siblings.Children with ODD may be verbally aggressive. They do not, however, exhibit physical aggression, which is typical of conduct disorder.

Furthermore, they must persist for more than six months and be deemed beyond the age, gender, and culture of a typical kid in order to qualify for the diagnosis. For children under the age of five, they must occur on the majority of days throughout a six-month period.

For children above the age of five, they must occur at least once every week for at least six months. If symptoms occur primarily in one environment, most typically at home, they are considered modest in intensity.

If the symptoms are present in two settings, they are classified as moderate, and if they appear in three or more settings, they are classified as severe.
These patterns of behavior cause difficulties at school or other social settings.

1.2 PREVALENCE OF ODD

ODD is a pattern of negative, rebellious, disobedient, and angry behavior that is one of the most common disorders from preschool to adulthood. This might involve frequent temper tantrums, excessive bickering with adults, refusing to obey rules, purposely upsetting people, being easily irritated, having an angry attitude, and engaging in vengeful behavior.

Children with ODD often develop symptoms between the ages of 6 and 8, however the illness may manifest in younger children as well. Symptoms might linger into the teenage years.The pooled prevalence is 3.6% up to the age of 18.

The frequency of oppositional defiant disorder ranges from one to eleven percent. The average prevalence is around 3%. Gender and age both influence the rate of the condition.ODD develops gradually and becomes noticeable in preschool, generally before the age of eight.However, it is quite unusual to appear beyond early adolescence.

Before adolescence, men had a greater incidence than females, by a ratio of 1.4 to one.Other research suggest a 2:1 ratio.The incidence in females seems to increase after puberty.Researchers observed that the overall prevalence of ODD across cultures remained consistent.

However, gender differences in diagnosis are only seen in Western nations. It is unclear if this reflects underlying differences in incidence or underdiagnosis among females. Physical abuse at home is a key predictor of diagnosis for girls alone, but emotional responsiveness of parents is a significant predictor of diagnosis for boys alone, which may have implications on gendered socialization and accepted gender roles.

Children from low-income households are more likely to be diagnosed with ODD. The relationship between low income and ODD diagnosis is straightforward in males, but it is more complicated in girls; the diagnosis is related with certain parenting practices such as physical punishment, which are linked to lower income homes. This gap may be related to a broader propensity for males and men to exhibit more externalized mental symptoms, whereas girls exhibit more internalized ones (such as self-harm or anorexia nervosa).

African Americans and Latinos are more likely to be diagnosed with ODD or other conduct disorders than non-Hispanic White kids experiencing the same symptoms, who are more likely to be labeled with ADHD. This has far-reaching consequences for understanding how racial prejudice influences how certain behaviors are seen and classified as rebellious or inattentive/hyperactive.

The prevalence of ODD and conduct disorder is much greater among foster youngsters. One poll in Norway indicated that 14 percent fit the criterion, whereas other investigations reported a frequency of up to 17 or even 29 percent.Low parental connection and parenting style are significant predictors of ODD symptoms.

Earlier ideas of ODD had greater diagnostic rates. When the condition was initially listed in the DSM-III, it had a 25% greater prevalence than when the DSM-IV altered the diagnostic criteria.The DSM-V makes further adjustments to the criteria, putting some features together to show that persons with ODD have both emotional and behavioral symptoms.

Furthermore, criteria were established to assist physicians in diagnosis due to the difficulties in determining whether the behaviors or other symptoms are directly connected to the condition or just a stage in a child's life.As a result, future research may show that prevalence decreased between the DSM-IV and the DSM-V.

Risk Factors For ODD

ODD, like other mental health problems, is caused by a mix of genetic, familial, and societal factors. Children with oppositional defiant disorder may have inherited chemical abnormalities in the brain, making them more susceptible to the disease.

Other risk factors for ODD are:

•inconsistent parental attention and discipline.

•Low socioeconomic status.

•Marital discord between parents
•Child Abuse or Neglect

•Brain injury.

Have a close family member with a mood disorder, behavior disorder, attention deficit disorder, or drug abuse problem.

Conditions that may coexist with ODD.

Children with ODD often have additional behavioral issues (comorbidities) that occur concurrently. Depression, anxiety, learning difficulties, communication issues, and attention deficit disorder (ADD) may all contribute to your child's rebellious behavior.

Children with oppositional defiant disorder may develop conduct disorder, which involves hostility towards others as well as more severe infractions of norms, including breaching the law.

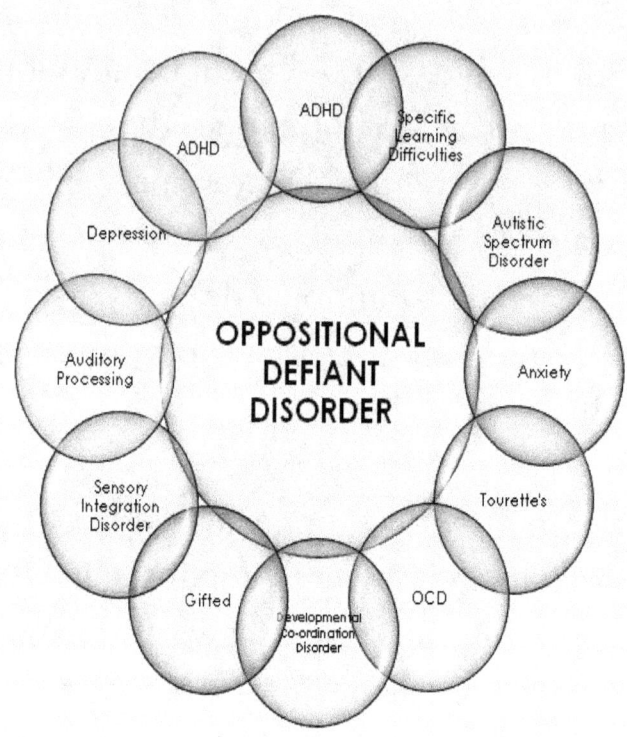

Related mental issues with ODD

1.3 CLINICAL ASSESSMENT AND DIAGNOSIS

To diagnose ODD, healthcare practitioners must have clinical expertise with the illness since there is no one test that can detect it. A child's behavioral habits are thoroughly evaluated in addition to obtaining a detailed medical history and physical examination.

A kid may be diagnosed with ODD if he or she meets the criteria outlined in the Diagnostic and Statistical Manual of Mental Disorders - Fifth Edition, or DSM-5.

Clinical assessment considers aspects such as:

general health of the youngster.

The frequency and severity of the behavior

Behavioral patterns fluctuate in various circumstances.

Other connected conditions that influence the child's psychological and intellectual development.

The latter is especially essential since it is fairly unusual to uncover co-existing mental illnesses in youngsters with ODD. It is also crucial to recognise these illnesses, since they may have a substantial impact on the child's prognosis if not addressed promptly.

DIAGNOSTIC CRITERIA

A youngster must present with at least four signs related to his or her mood, behavior, or vindictiveness. In terms of mood, a kid is evaluated to see if he or she is often resentful or angry, easily frustrated, and/or fast to fly off the handle. Argumentative attitudes with figures of authority, refusal to comply with demands (in a spirit of defiance), willful efforts to irritate others, and blaming others for one's own wrongdoing and/or errors are some of the behavioral factors to be considered.

A youngster who has been vengeful or spiteful at least twice in the last six months fulfills the vindictiveness criteria for ODD.

It is critical to distinguish between what is developmentally appropriate for a child's age and ODD. In children under the age of five, the behavioral requirements should be satisfied for at least six months and on the majority of days during that time.

Children aged 5 and above should demonstrate ODD-related symptoms at least once per week for at least six months. These criteria serve as a diagnostic guide for determining the disorder's acceptable age-related frequency.

They should be combined with other characteristics to assess if the behavioral pattern is unusual from a cultural, gender, or developmental standpoint.

1.4 THE EFFECT OF ODD ON CHILD DEVELOPMENT AND FAMILY DYNAMICS.

Oppositional Defiant Disorder (ODD) has a substantial impact on both child development and family interactions, presenting issues that must be understood and addressed psychologically. ODD is defined by persistent behaviors of defiance, disobedience, and animosity towards authority figures. This article investigates how ODD influences child development and family relations, as well as psychologists' roles in treating these issues.

First and foremost, ODD may inhibit healthy child development. Children with ODD frequently suffer with emotional control, making it difficult to build healthy interactions with peers and authoritative figures. Their disruptive behavior might jeopardize academic achievement and social integration, lowering their self-esteem and general well-being. Psychologists play an important role in screening and diagnosing ODD, as well as delivering personalized therapies to help children grow emotionally and behaviorally.

Secondly, ODD has a significant impact on family interactions. The continual disobedience and conflict that comes with ODD may strain parent-child relationships and impede family function. Parents may feel frustrated, guilty, or stressed when controlling their child's behavior, which may lead to family problems. Siblings may feel ignored or overshadowed by the frequent focus on the kid with ODD. Psychologists collaborate with families to improve communication, adopt good parenting practices, and provide a supportive atmosphere that promotes the child's growth.

Furthermore, untreated ODD might have long-term implications if not addressed. Without adequate help, children with ODD are more likely to develop conduct disorder and other behavioral issues in adolescence and adulthood.

These people may struggle to sustain work, build stable relationships, and engage in prosocial behavior. Early intervention by psychologists is critical in minimizing the development of ODD symptoms and minimizing possible harmful repercussions later in life.

Finally, Oppositional Defiant Disorder has a profound influence on both child development and family interactions, providing issues that psychologists must address on several levels.

Understanding the complexity of ODD and its repercussions enables psychologists to offer thorough evaluations, treatments, and support systems that encourage good results for both the child and their family. It is feasible to handle the obstacles offered by ODD while still promoting healthy growth within the family unit.

CHAPTER 2: EVIDENCE-BASED TREATMENTS FOR ODD

2.1 BEHAVIOURAL PARENT TRAINING FOR ODD.

Behavioral parent training (BPT) teaches parents how to use behavior management and disciplinary techniques to extend therapy from the therapist's office to the home, addressing a broad range of problem behaviors.

BPT programmes are intended to educate parents about ADHD and offer them methods for improving the parent-child connection, reducing problem behaviors, and increasing desirable behaviors.

Nearly all BPT programmes are based on the Hanf two-stage model (Reitman and McMahon, 2013), which encourages parents to concentrate on instilling positivity in parent-child interactions in order to create a framework for successful punishment.

BPT programmes are generally delivered in 8 to 16 group or individual sessions, each directed by a qualified therapist. Using a collaborative approach, the clinician chats with parents about the particular issues in their household and assists them in implementing the BPT procedures to address these challenges.

The sessions typically cover the following skills: labeled praise, positive reinforcement, special parent-child time, active ignoring, effective instructions, time out for noncompliance and aggression, house rule development and enforcement, token economies, effective home-school communication, and problem-solving techniques for future difficulties.

BPT has been proven to be successful in lowering parent-rated disruptive behaviors, aggressiveness, and ADHD symptoms, as well as enhancing child compliance, parental discipline skills, and parenting self-efficacy (review by Chronis et al., 2004).

BPT programmes have been tailored to address the requirements of certain groups, such as single mothers, moms with ADHD or depression, and families facing transportation challenges (Evans et al., 2018b).

In summary,Behavioral parent training has been shown successful in a variety of contexts, forms, processes, intensities, and durations. When prioritizing treatment aims and creating parent goals for success, the context of parent training, which includes family routines, culture, educational background, socioeconomic situation, and stress level, must be taken into account.

To get long-term results, you must plan for maintenance and generalization and educate parents how to assess the success of the approaches they use with their kid. ACT may be an effective technique for parents who suffer from chronic stress or depression, which impairs their capacity to learn or follow the methods taught during parent training.

2.2 COGNITIVE-BEHAVIORAL THERAPY (CBT) APPROACHES TO ODD

Cognitive Behavioural Therapy is a kind of talk therapy that may assist with mental health issues. Dr. Ellen Braaten's CBT Snapshot series provides an overview of how CBT is used to treat a variety of mental and behavioral health conditions.

Dan, a 7-year-old boy, was regarded by his parents as continuously disobedient. He was quickly irritated and usually annoying to others. He regularly lost his anger, usually over little issues like not having the "right" cereal for breakfast. He seldom finished his schoolwork and never did the duties that his parents assigned him. With the exception of not doing his schoolwork, he had few issues at school. In fact, when questioned why he acted this way at home, he said, "Because my parents are always on my back."

Dan was diagnosed with oppositional defiant disorder. His behaviors are typical of youngsters with this illness, as he exhibited negative attitudes, confrontational behavior, and disobedience. Children with Conduct Disorder and ODD on the other hand, engage in more extreme forms of aggressiveness that may result in bodily injury to themselves and others.

Tom's parents were concerned that he was moving in this route, since he had lately grown more deceptive and took money from a classmate's bag. Tom's parents sought therapy from a psychologist who used Cognitive Behaviour Therapy (CBT), which involved educating the parents how to change their behavior to discourage Tom's rebellious behavior while also supporting Tom's proper behavior.

Tom's therapist employed a mix of family meetings, parent-child meetings, and individual sessions with Tom. During Tom's sessions, the therapist would have him practice more adaptive methods to assist him establish a feeling of mastery and achievement in settings with family or friends. Tom realized that he might be less violent in a therapeutic atmosphere.

Tom's therapist also saw that Tom's self-esteem needed to improve before he could make good changes, therefore raising self-esteem was one of their objectives. In terms of the parent-child interaction, Tom's therapist was aware that strong physical and verbal punishment may lead to more aggressive and deviant behavior, and he was concerned that their parenting style was exacerbating the problem. Thus, throughout his time with Tom's parents, the therapist assisted them in substituting harsh, punitive parenting tactics with milder discipline measures.

Overall, CBT therapy has been shown to be fairly helpful in treating disruptive behavior problems. Treatment that combines parent training with problem-solving skills training for children is very successful. In fact, combining the two treatments has been demonstrated to be more beneficial than any therapy alone, especially in children aged 7 and above. These programmes often have the following features:

An emphasis on the child's cognitive processes in interpersonal connections. During therapy, the kid is taught to address interpersonal difficulties in a step-by-step manner.

An focus on enhancing prosocial behaviors via modeling or reinforcement.

Use games, tales, and exercises to improve cognitive problem-solving abilities. As treatment proceeds, these abilities are more used in real-world settings at school and at home.

An active therapy technique in which the therapist models proper behavior, teaches adaptive skills, and provides feedback on both good and negative behaviors.

2.3 ADDITIONAL CONSIDERED THERAPIES.

•Parental-child interaction treatment (PCIT)

This treatment for children with ODD involves real-time parenting coaching offered by a therapist who observes participants in a playroom via one-way glass.

The therapist communicates with the parent utilizing a wireless in-ear speaker. In this environment, the therapist may see the parent-child relationship in real time, rather than depending on the parents' memory of earlier experiences.

A study Trusted Source comprising 81 Norwegian families with children aged 2 to 7 years indicated that the PCIT group had a higher decrease in behavior issues than the individuals who received standard therapy.

•Collaborative problem solving (CPS).

CPS recognises that persons with ODD lack the abilities to get along, not the desire to do so. Rather than imposing their will on others or walking away entirely, CPS members are taught to strike a balance via discussion and compromise.

A 2004 studyTrusted Source of 47 children with ODD found that CPS achieved effects that were either equivalent or superior to parent training.

•Peer Group Therapy

This sort of social skills treatment teaches persons with ODD how to interact more effectively with their peers. The idea is to promote pleasant encounters over aggressive ones. This treatment is most effective when performed in a natural context, such as school.

2.4 MEDICATION OPTIONS AND CONSIDERATIONS FOR ODD

Medication may assist persons with ODD manage their comorbid diseases. For example, stimulant medicine may alleviate the difficulties produced by ADHD symptoms, hence reducing ODD symptoms.

ODD patients may benefit from the following medications:

•Stimulant Medications

Stimulant medication is often used to treat ADHD, and multiple studies have linked these drugs to improved ODD symptoms in children with ADHD.

Stimulants utilized include methylphenidate (MPH) and mixed amphetamine salts (MAS).

•Atomoxetine (ATX)

ATX is a nonstimulant ADHD drug that may help reduce ODD symptoms. It's unclear if ATX helps for ODD or whether it improves ODD symptoms indirectly by lowering ADHD symptoms.

•Atypical antipsychotics.

Risperidone (Risperdal) is an atypical antipsychotic that is used cautiously to treat ODD aggressiveness.

Doctors may prescribe it when treatment and stimulant medicine have failed and the individual with ODD is suffering from severe side effects as a result of the ODD symptoms.

Risperidone is considered a last-resort therapy since it might cause potentially severe metabolic, hormonal, and neurological abnormalities.

•Self-Care Strategies

While therapy is the primary treatment for ODD, and medication may sometimes assist, there are other self-care methods that can help to alleviate symptoms.

Mindfulness is a strong skill for regulating emotions and achieving tranquility. Mindfulness is the discipline of focusing your attention on the present moment and letting your thoughts pass without participating in them. Meditation is only one of many techniques to practice awareness.

Try stress-reduction techniques to alleviate ODD symptoms. Several concepts include:

•listening to music

•Talking with a buddy

•Eating a healthy diet.

•Exercise frequently.

•Have a nice chuckle

•Prioritizing sleep.

Living with ODD is doable with the correct assistance. If you suspect you have ODD, speak with a healthcare or mental health expert to rule out alternative reasons for your symptoms.

CHAPTER 3: PRACTICAL STRATEGIES FOR HANDLING ODD BEHAVIORS

3.1 SETTING CLEAR AND CONSISTENT BOUNDARIES

Children with ODD benefit from having clear and consistent rules that offer structure and limits. When setting rules, make them explicit, age-appropriate, and simple to grasp. Clearly convey the rules to your kid and make sure they understand the consequences of not following them.

Enforcing these standards requires consistent application. It is critical for all carers to be on the same page and consistently apply the regulations.

Inconsistency may create uncertainty and intensify rebellious behavior.

Remember to maintain reasonable expectations and be prepared to continually repeat the guidelines over time.

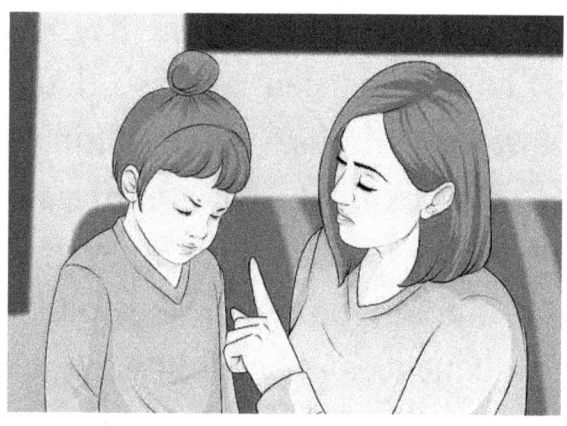

Setting of boundaries help children   with ODD

Tips for Setting Clear and Consistent Rules

•Set guidelines that are clear, detailed, and age-appropriate.

•Communicate the rules to your kid, and make sure they understand the consequences of not following them.

•Enforce the guidelines consistently and make sure all carers are on the same page.
•Set realistic expectations and be prepared to regularly enforce the rules over time.

3.2 POSITIVE REINFORCEMENT AND REWARDS.

Positive reinforcement and prizes may be useful techniques for promoting desirable behaviors and motivating youngsters with

ODD. Recognise and applaud your child's efforts and successes, no matter how minor. This boosts their self-esteem and encourages good behavior.

Consider developing a reward system in which your kid gets privileges or modest incentives for completing certain objectives or according to defined regulations. This might create a feeling of organization and drive. Make sure the incentives are relevant to your kid and age appropriate.

Tips for Positive Reinforcement and Incentives.

•Recognise and applaud your child's efforts and successes, no matter how minor.

•Implement a reward system in which your kid receives privileges or tiny prizes for achieving certain objectives or according to defined norms.

•Make sure the incentives are relevant to your kid and age appropriate.

•Implementing the stated parenting practices can help to establish a more positive and supportive atmosphere for your kid with ODD.

Remember that receiving professional treatment and working with mental health specialists is critical for properly controlling ODD.

3.3 EFFECTIVE COMMUNICATION

When working with a kid with ODD, effective communication is vital. It is critical to have a calm and courteous demeanor even in difficult times. Avoid power clashes by focusing on active listening and understanding your child's point of view.

Use "I" expressions to communicate your sentiments and worries without accusing or criticizing your youngster. This may assist to de-escalate tensions and foster open communication. Encourage your children to communicate their feelings and opinions in a safe and healthy way.

Tips for Effective CommunicationMaintain a cool and courteous demeanor, especially in difficult times.Avoid power battles and prioritize active listening.Use "I" expressions to communicate your sentiments and worries without accusing or criticizing your youngster.Encourage your kid to share their feelings and views in a safe and productive way.

3.4 PROFESSIONAL INTERVENTION.

Parenting a kid with Oppositional Defiant Disorder (ODD) presents unique problems. However, with the correct tactics and assistance, you can successfully regulate their behavior and establish healthy connections. In this part, we will look at three important parenting practices for children with ODD: creating clear and consistent rules, effective communication skills, and positive reinforcement and incentives.

When to Consider Professional Intervention

Parents should seek professional help if their child's ODD symptoms seriously disrupt their daily life, relationships, and general well-being. Some indicators that may suggest the need for professional assistance are:

•Persistent and severe behavioral issues that are challenging to handle at home, school, or in social situations.

•Ongoing disagreements with authority officials, such as parents, teachers, or carers.

•Aggressive or aggressive behavior towards others or oneself.

•Frequent and severe angry outbursts that are out of proportion to the circumstances.

•Failure to respond to parental tactics and treatments.

If you observe any of these indicators or are concerned about your child's behavior, you should speak with a mental health expert. They may do a thorough examination to see if the behaviors fulfill the criteria for ODD or if there are any coexisting illnesses that need treatment.

Types of Professional Help Available

There are several mental health specialists that may provide assistance and therapy to children with ODD. These professions could include:

•**Child and Adolescent Psychiatrists:** These medical professionals focus on identifying and treating mental health issues in children and adolescents. They can help with medication management if required.

•**Psychologists** : are educated to evaluate and treat behavioral and emotional disorders. They may provide treatment and assistance in developing techniques to control ODD symptoms.

•**Licensed Clinical Social Workers (LCSWs)** :are trained to provide counseling and treatment. They may work with both the kid and the family to alleviate ODD symptoms and enhance family relationships.

•**Therapists or Counselors:** These professionals may have a variety of degrees and certifications, including Licenced Professional Counselors (LPC) and Marriage and Family Therapists (MFT). They may provide treatment and assistance to children with ODD and their families.

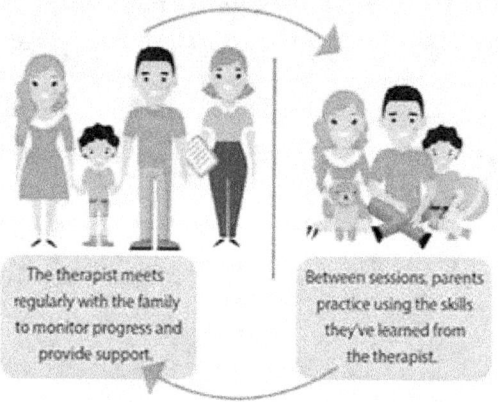

What parents can expect in behavior therapy

Parents typically attend 8-16 sessions with a therapist and learn strategies to help their child. Sessions may involve groups or individual families.

The therapist meets regularly with the family to monitor progress and provide support.

Between sessions, parents practice using the skills they've learned from the therapist.

Counseling and therapies helps children with ODD

Collaboration with Mental Health Professionals.

•Collaboration between parents and mental health experts is critical for successfully treating ODD. When meeting with a mental health professional, parents should:

•Provide pertinent facts about their child's behavior, including specific instances and trends.

•Please include any paperwork or assessments completed by teachers or other experts.

•Be upfront and honest about their personal issues, struggles, and therapeutic objectives.

•Actively engage in treatment sessions and implement the prescribed tactics and interventions.

•Maintain frequent contact with the mental health professional to review progress and resolve any issues.

Remember that seeking professional assistance is not a sign of failure as a parent, but rather a proactive move towards helping your child's health. Collaboration with mental health specialists may assist parents in developing successful methods and providing the essential support to enable children with ODD flourish.

Resources and Additional Support

When dealing with Oppositional Defiant Disorder (ODD) in children, it is critical to have access to resources and extra help. These sites may provide parents with support, knowledge, and a feeling of community as they navigate the difficulties of parenting a kid with ODD.Some helpful resources are listed below:

Books and Literature About ODD

Books and literature may provide parents with useful knowledge and help in understanding and managing their children's ODD. These materials provide insights, tactics, and practical guidance from industry leaders.

Books may help you understand and manage children's ODD behaviors. Remember that each kid is unique, so speaking with a mental health expert may help you adjust techniques to your child's individual requirements.

Support Groups and Online Communities

Connecting with people who are going through similar circumstances may help parents feel more supported and understood. Support groups and online forums for ODD may be a great source of emotional support, information exchange, and practical help.

These communities enable parents to connect with others who are having similar issues and exchange methods that have been effective for them. Some online communities and support groups include the following:

Oppositional Defiant Disorder Support Group.

Parents of children with oppositional defiant disorder should be Participating in these support groups and online forums may help parents feel less lonely while also providing a forum for discussing problems and learning from the experiences of others.

CHAPTER 4: PROMOTING RESILIENCE AND LONG-TERM SUCCESS

4.1 STRENGTHENING PARENT-CHILD RELATIONSHIPS

Oppositional Defiant Disorder (ODD) may provide substantial issues for both children and their parents. However, it is feasible to assist children with ODD in developing resilience and efficiently managing their symptoms.

In this part, we will look at three major tactics for developing resilience in children with ODD: supporting emotional control, teaching problem-solving abilities, and fostering good coping mechanisms.

Encouraging Emotional Regulation.

Emotional control is a crucial ability for children with ODD to acquire. It entails recognising and efficiently regulating their emotions in a healthy and suitable way. Parents may help their children regulate their emotions by:

•**Encouraging open communication:** Provide a secure and nonjudgmental environment for your youngster to share their emotions. Listen actively and validate their experiences.

•**Teaching relaxation techniques:** Use deep breathing exercises or mindfulness activities to assist your kid calm down during times of emotional discomfort.

•Modeling emotional control: Set a good example for others by practicing healthy emotional management yourself. Show your youngster how to express and manage emotions in a positive manner.

Teaching Problem Solving Skills

Children with ODD often struggle with problem-solving skills, which may result in frequent disagreements and demanding behaviors. Parents may help their children handle challenging situations more effectively by teaching them effective problem-solving skills. Here are some strategies to consider.

•Break down difficulties: Help your youngster divide complicated problems into smaller, more manageable chunks.

This may make problem-solving seem less daunting.

•**Explore other ideas:** Encourage your kid to brainstorm many solutions to an issue, taking into account both the advantages and disadvantages of each choice.

•**Evaluate the implications:** Help your youngster realize the possible repercussions of their behavior. Discuss the implications of alternative options and help them make educated judgements.

Promoting Healthy Coping Mechanisms

Promoting good coping techniques is critical for children with ODD to manage stress and frustration constructively. Here are some ways to encourage good coping mechanisms:

•**Encourage physical exercise:** Regular physical activity may assist to decrease stress and enhance overall health. Encourage your kid to engage in activities that he or she enjoys, such as athletics, dance, or yoga.

•Encourage your kid to express their feelings via creative activities such as painting, music, or writing. These outlets provide healthy avenues for people to absorb and express their emotions.

•**Teach relaxation methods:** To assist your kid cope with stress and anxiety, provide strategies like progressive muscle relaxation or guided visualization.

Parents who concentrate on these tactics may play an important role in developing resilience in children with ODD. It's vital to remember that every kid is different, and what works for one may not work for another. Patience, consistency, and a supportive environment are critical for helping children with ODD build resilience and flourish. Visit our pages on impulse control disorders and conduct disorder versus oppositional defiant disorder to learn more about these conditions.

4.2   PROMOTING   SOCIAL CONNECTIONS

Social ties are critical to the growth and well-being of children with ODD. Encouraging good connections with classmates, family members, and other supportive people may help them enhance their social and emotional abilities. Participating in activities that encourage collaboration, empathy, and cooperation may improve their behavior and overall resilience.

Parents may help their children form social relationships by immersing them in organized activities like sports, clubs, or community programmes. These activities allow the youngster to engage with others who have similar interests and create a feeling of belonging. It is critical to monitor these social contacts and give assistance as needed to ensure that they stay pleasant and helpful.

4.3 CREATING A SUPPORTIVE AND UNDERSTANDING ENVIRONMENT

When it comes to assisting children with Oppositional Defiant Disorder (ODD), a supportive atmosphere is crucial. By creating a supportive and understanding environment, parents may help manage ODD symptoms and promote good behavior.

In this part, we will look at three important components of building a supportive environment for children with ODD: educating family members and carers, fostering social connections, and practicing self-care as parents.

Educating Family and Carers

One of the first stages in building a supportive environment for a kid with ODD is to educate family members and carers about the condition. Everyone involved may benefit from correct understanding of ODD, its signs and symptoms, and treatment techniques. This information contributes to promoting empathy, patience, and good communication within the family unit.

Family members and carers should be encouraged to participate in support groups, courses, or seek professional help to improve their knowledge of ODD. By arming themselves with information, parents can give consistent and appropriate assistance to the youngster.

4.4 PRACTICE SELF-CARE FOR PARENTS

Caring for a kid with ODD may be cognitively and emotionally taxing. As a result, it is critical for parents to prioritize their own health and engage in self-care. Self-care enables parents to be more patient, empathetic, and resilient when faced with problems.

Self-care for parents may take many forms, including indulging in hobbies, getting help from friends or support groups, and taking time to rest and recharge. It's vital to remember that self-care isn't selfish; it's an essential part of being a good carer. Parents who prioritize their own physical and emotional well-being may better help their kid with ODD.

Creating a supportive environment requires a joint effort by all family members and carers engaged in the child's life. Parents may assist and understand their child's well-being by learning about ODD, promoting social connections, and practicing self-care.

A supportive environment, when combined with expert assistance and suitable management measures, may significantly contribute to children's resilience and healthy development with ODD.

SUMMARY AND CONCLUSIONS

"Oppositional Defiant Disorder: Possible Treatments and Strategies for Overcoming it in Children" explores the complexity of dealing with oppositional behavior in children. It is authored by a psychologist and provides a complete review of evidence-based therapies like cognitive-behavioral therapy, parent training programmes, and pharmaceutical choices.

The book emphasizes the value of early intervention and a multidisciplinary approach that includes parents, educators, and mental health specialists. Practical ways for enhancing parent-child communication, establishing definitive boundaries, and encouraging positive reinforcement are discussed. The authors also investigate the influence of environmental variables and genetics in the development of oppositional behaviors.

Finally, "Oppositional Defiant Disorder: Possible Treatments and how to Overcome it in Children" offers vital insights and practical help to parents, educators, and therapists dealing with ODD.

By adopting personalized therapies and creating a supportive environment, children with ODD may develop better coping skills and enhance their overall well-being.

www.ingramcontent.com/pod-product-compliance
Lightning Source LLC
Chambersburg PA
CBHW071102290526
45795CB00004B/1619